CBD And Hemp Oil

A Simple Patient's Healing Guide To Using CBD And Hemp Oil To Cure Physical And Psychological Pain And Illness

Ryan Archer

Table of Contents

Introduction 1

Chapter One: What Can CBD Do For You? 6

Chapter Two: What Others Say 20

Chapter Three: Hemp Oil 26

Chapter Four: Which Is For Me? 32

Chapter Five: How To Get It 36

Chapter Six: Legal Information 42

Wellness 46

Conclusion 49

© Copyright 2018 - All rights reserved.

It is not legal to reproduce, duplicate, or transmit any part of this document in either electronic means or in printed format. Recording of this publication is strictly prohibited and any storage of this document is not allowed unless with written permission from the publisher except for the use of brief quotations in a book review.

Introduction

I am sure you have heard a thing or two about cannabidiol or CBD. CBD is found in the cannabis plant and has become a very popular supplement. It has been introduced as a great option for medicinal purposes and though its use is increasing, it will probably take some time to become more mainstream. The reason for this is due to many misconceptions surrounding cannabis, as well as the stigma that many societies have against it and its usage being illegal in many parts of the world.

My guess is that you are reading this book because you have many questions about CBD and hemp oil. You have an open mind about their use but are still unsure of a few things. In this book, I will discuss the benefits of CBD and hemp oil and will further dispel a few prevalent notions about CBD and hemp oil.

Firstly, one must remember that the use of cannabis itself is by no means a new phenomenon. While the Western World is increasing funding toward research for a better understanding of the plant, it has been used in abundance on the Indian subcontinent for thousands of years. It has been used for medicinal purposes, although this usage has often been overshadowed by recreational use. As a result, cannabis has negative connotations attached to it. This is what may have caused you to approach CBD and hemp oil with trepidation.

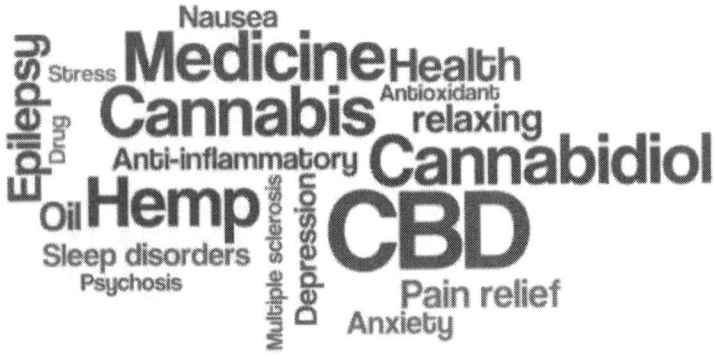

Medicinal cannabis in the form of CBD and hemp can provide tremendous benefits. You may have heard many of these terms associated with medicinal cannabis but are unsure of what the connection is. Don't fret! Read on!

Image Credit: Shutterstock.com

So let us first have a better understanding of the root of it all.

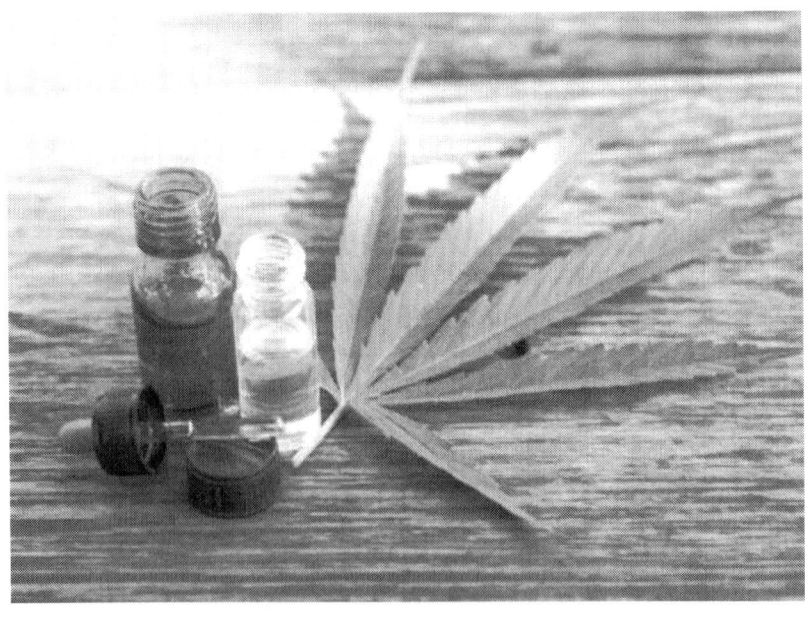

The cannabis plant is now being used for medicinal purposes all over the U.S.

Image Credit: Shutterstock.com

Cannabaceae is the name of the family of plants from which cannabis comes. In simple English, this family of plants is known as the hemp family. From the plants of the hemp family come many chemicals called cannabinoids. Of the hundreds of cannabinoids, cannabidiol (CBD) is the one that seems to offer the most benefits for the human body.

Briefly, here are some of the benefits that CBD Oil has:

- Alleviating the symptoms of social or psychological disorders
- Alleviating physical pain
- Aiding in the treatment of serious illnesses

So where exactly do we find CBD? CBD is actually found all throughout the cannabis plant -- and as a result, it is easy to withdraw and sell in abundance. One of the worries that many people have about using hemp-based products is that they do not want to smoke to get the benefits. The prevalent image of cannabis has been of the plant rolled up in a paper and smoked like a cigarette. But for consuming CBD, this does not have to be the case. As a product, CBD can be consumed in a variety of ways: through a pill or capsule, as a suppository, or even as a chewing gum!

You may still be skeptical of CBD due to the stigma surrounding the cannabis plant. One thing to remember is that this stigma actually has nothing to do with cannabis or hemp, but is rather to do with marijuana. So what is the main difference between CBD and marijuana? The answer is that marijuana contains tetrahydrocannabinol or THC. THC is another cannabinoid that is found throughout the cannabis plant, but unlike CBD, it has psychoactive effects. These psychoactive effects produce the euphoria or "high" that one gets from smoking marijuana. It is for this reason that marijuana is looked upon as purely recreational and even as dangerous. It is because of this that it remains illegal in many areas of the world.

Though both CBD and THC are found in the cannabis plant, it is important to distinguish between the two. One should note that CBD is *not* a psychoactive drug and the effects that one would get from smoking marijuana recreationally will not be an issue when consuming CBD. In the United States, scientists have noted that the cannabis plant can cause users to become addicted. However, with contemporary studies learning about the benefits of the plant, there is a decreasing stigma and an increase in advocacy for using the plant for medicinal purposes.

So, how exactly does CBD affect the body? What about cannabis makes it useful for medicinal purposes? To answer this, you need to have an understanding of the endocannabinoid system. The endocannabinoid system was found when researchers wanted to discover how cannabis worked on our bodies. It is made up of cannabinoid receptors, which are found throughout the human body. Two of the main cannabinoid receptors are cannabinoid receptor type 1 (CB1) and cannabinoid receptor type 2 (CB2). CB1 is found in the central and peripheral nervous system. The central nervous system consists of the brain and the spinal cord; the peripheral nervous system extends to nerves affecting the muscles, taste, touch, the heart, and the digestive system. These receptors help to heal the body and can be stimulated by cannabinoids like CBD that are found in the cannabis plant.

You now have a general overview of CBD and of cannabis. But you probably still have a few questions regarding the medicinal use of CBD. Do you need CBD? Is CBD going to help a particular ailment or ailments that you have? We will discuss this in the next chapter.

Please note that the contents of this book are based upon the author's research. Always consult a medical professional before purchasing and/or consuming CBD, hemp oil or any cannabis-related product for medicinal purposes.

Chapter One: What Can CBD Do For You?

By now, we have hopefully dispelled any false notions you had regarding cannabis and CBD oil. You will now learn about how CBD can be a great medicine for a variety of ailments.

Acne

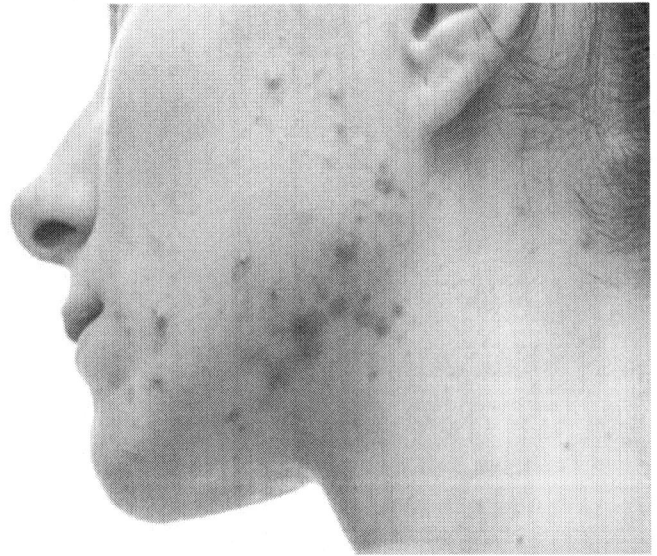

Acne is one of the most common skin diseases.

Image Credit: Shutterstock.com

Acne is something many of us deal with -- although we wish we didn't! Acne is a skin disease that usually occurs during adolescence but that can continue for many years to come. Many people will do whatever it takes to be rid of acne. They try various creams, ointments, and even make changes to their diet in hope of ridding themselves of acne. However, it's unlikely that many people have tried CBD oil as an acne cure, although studies have found that it can fight acne.

Acne is caused by the buildup of lipids (oil) which eventually leads to pimples, scars, blackheads, and whiteheads on the skin. To understand how CBD oil works to minimize acne, one must understand the concept of the endocannabinoid system. Endocannabinoids are lipid-based and connect to cannabinoid receptors. A study shows that when CBD oil provides calcium to be the body, which hinders the continuous development of lipids.

Feeling Anxious?

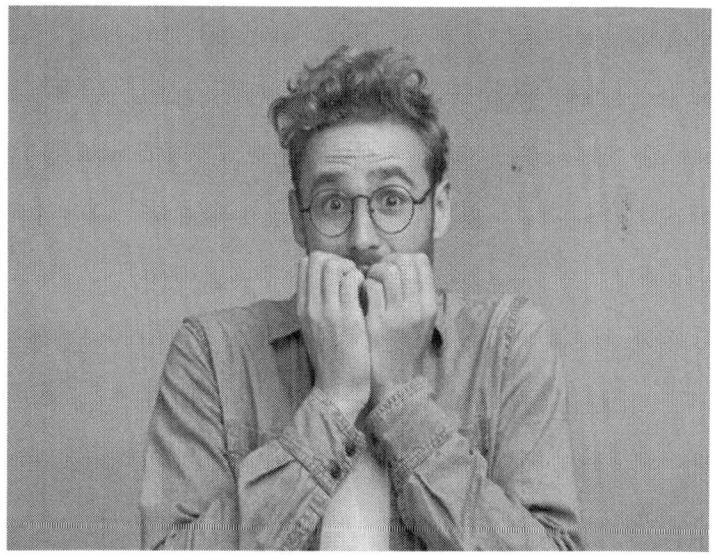

CBD is often used to help treat the anxiety.

Image Credit: Shutterstock.com

Anxiety is a growing problem. Smoking cannabis has often been looked at a way to treat anxiety, but due to the stigma surrounding marijuana, this notion has been dismissed for quite some time. However, more recent studies have validated the possibility of CBD oil as a treatment for anxiety. One must remember that marijuana is high in THC, which can agitate anxiety symptoms; CBD oil, however, has a very little or no THC and can therefore relax the nervous system. With the high levels of THC found in marijuana, an individual may be susceptible to paranoia and increased fear when smoking marijuana. The low THC in CBD oil, conversely, is able to decrease and even eliminate such irrational fears. As with medical cannabis as a whole, CBD is slowly but surely gaining popularity as an option for fighting anxiety.

When You Are Feeling Down

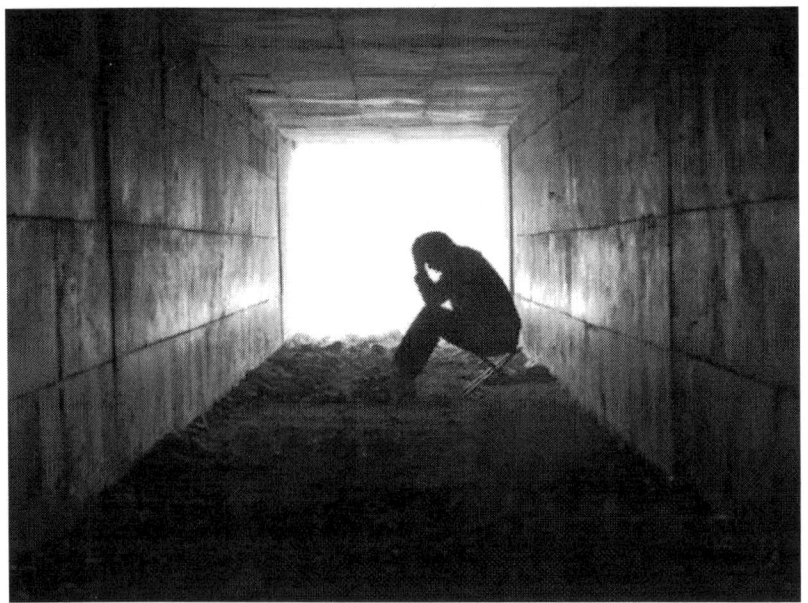

One of the most common and detrimental psychological disorders is depression.

Image Credit: Shutterstock.com

But of course, the usefulness of cannabis does not end with anxiety. There are many mental and psychological disorders that can be treated with CBD oil. Perhaps even more so than anxiety, depression is a growing phenomenon and affects everyone from adolescents to older adults. Before deciding to treat yourself with CBD oil, it is imperative to find out if you actually have depression. Many people are uninformed about mental illness as a whole and depression in particular. They will often say things like, "I'm depressed now" or "That's depressing" without knowing how depression truly feels. Depression is not simply feeling sad. However, if you have persistent feelings of sadness, you should consult a medical professional to determine whether or not you actually have depression. Only if you do should you look into using CBD oil to help treat your depression symptoms.

Studies have been conducted on mice to test the effectiveness of CBD oil in treating depression. After hyperactive mice were injected with CBD oil, their hyperactivity decreased within half an hour. Hyperactivity is one of the symptoms of both anxiety and depression in human beings. A study at the Al Ain campus of United Arab Emirates University found that black pepper can help fight depression. Black pepper is rich in beta-caryophyllene which is also found in *Cannabis sativa*, from which CBD oil is extracted. At the University of Buffalo, a study found that the chronic stress humans experience decreases the production of endocannabinoids, which can lead to depression. CBD oil can help replace these lost endocannabinoids.

A specific form of depression is postpartum depression, which occurs after childbirth. Doctors have often prescribed antidepressants or recommended therapy to fight against postpartum depression. As stated before, CBD oil has been found to lower stress, anxiety, and feelings of sadness, which makes it a potential treatment for postpartum depression. However, as of this writing, little conducive research has been conducted on the effects of taking CBD oil while breastfeeding a child, so it is always best to seek the advice of a medical professional before taking it or any other treatment.

Arthritis

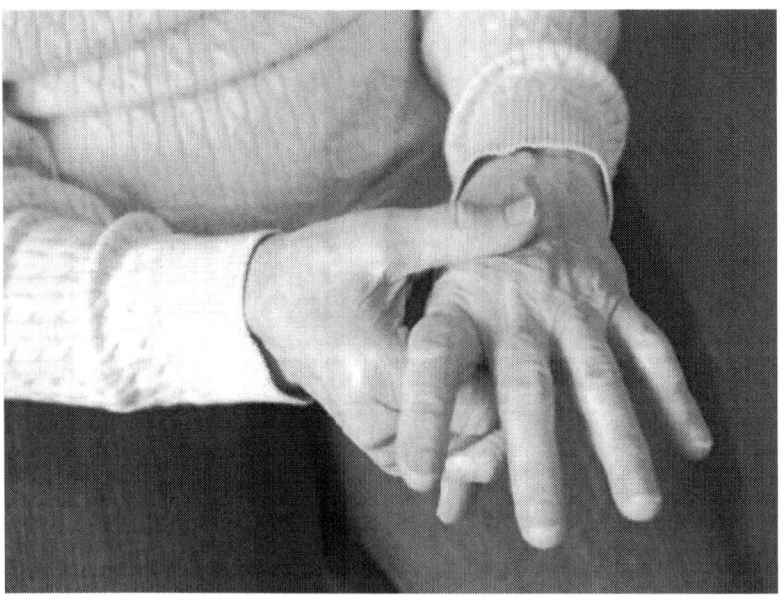

Arthritis can cause joint pain and stiffness.

Image Credit: Shutterstock.com

There are over one hundred types of arthritis diseases, and contrary to popular belief, arthritis can be found in people of all ages. One type of arthritis is rheumatoid arthritis, which causes inflammation and pain in the joints. While it has been slow in gaining acceptance, cannabis has been used to treat rheumatoid arthritis for quite a while. CBD can be applied as an oil or as a cream onto the skin for treating rheumatoid arthritis. CBD oil can reduce inflammation and, as a result, reduce the pain caused by rheumatoid arthritis.

The Heart

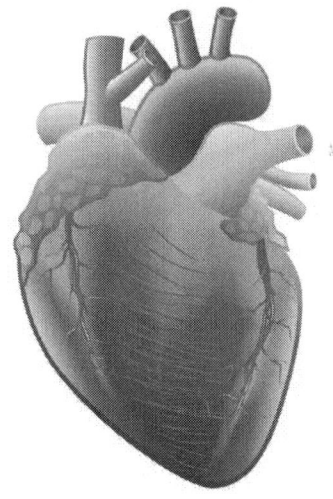

Heart disease is the number one cause of death of adults in the US.

Image Credit: Shutterstock.com

According to statistics provided by the American Heart Association, heart disease is the number one cause of death of adults in the United States. Where does cannabis come into play in fighting heart disease? Professor Alexander Stokes at the University of Hawaii believes that cannabis can improve the strength of the heart. When an individual is suffering from heart disease, the heart pumps blood at a slower rate. Professor Stokes believes that cannabis can help pump the blood more frequently. One of the cellular receptors present in our peripheral nervous system as well as our central nervous system is TRPV1 which can cause heart failure. Stimulating cannabinoid receptors such as CB1 and CB2 may be able to fight TRPV1 and therefore improve heart conditions. Cannabinoids have the same qualities as spices and peppers, which are known to stave off TRPV1.

Scientists, doctors, and medical professionals continue to study the effects of cannabis on the cardiovascular system. Some studies have shown that while cannabis can increase the heart rate (as found by Professor Stokes), an increased heart rate can lead to other problems, such as heart attack or stroke. As research on the relationship between cannabis and the cardiovascular system is still being done, it is always best to consult your doctor on whether or not you should implement the use of CBD oil to improve a heart condition.

I Need Some Sleep!

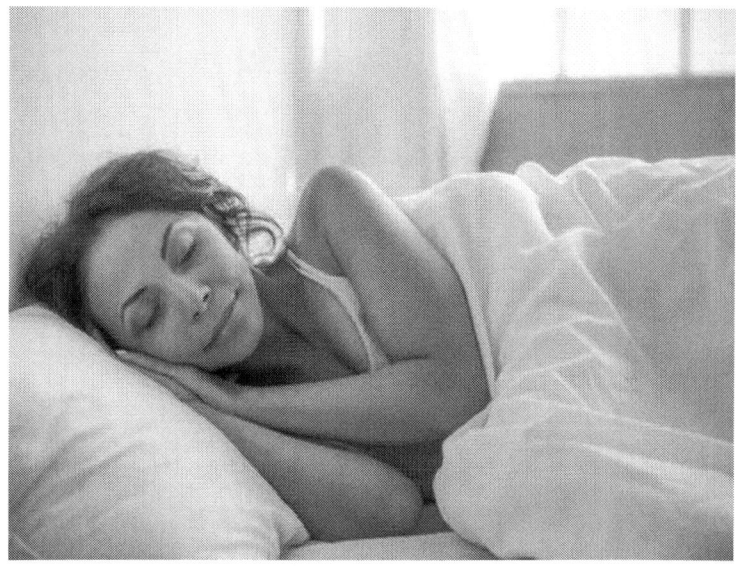

Sleep is crucial for overall wellness.

Image Credit: Shutterstock.com

We could all use a good night's sleep! Sleep is essential for maintaining overall health and preventing future diseases. Regardless of what category of illness you may *already* have, sleep is a necessary factor in treating the illness. Sleep is almost like the part of the prescription which is not written down -- because it should be a given! But many people have difficulty sleeping well even if they are feeling fatigued. So what can you do to improve your sleep? Can cannabis play a role in improving your sleeping patterns?

Before actually falling asleep, your body has to prepare to progress from being awake to being asleep. Before falling into a deep sleep, many people are asleep but can still easily be awoken. Eventually, a deep sleep is achieved. The goal is to remain in a deep sleep for as long as is needed to have an effective rest. During a deep sleep, individuals may experience rapid eye movement or REM. The exact purpose of REM is debated, but most scientists agree that it has something to do with dreaming and memory-processing.

So how does cannabis come into play with the different stages of sleep? Studies have shown that using cannabis can decrease length of the REM stage of sleep. Cannabis users have been shown to have difficulty recalling their dreams. As a result, if we assume that REM sleep benefits the human body, you would want to regulate your use of cannabis and ensure that it does not affect your REM sleep. However, cannabis is very popular among people who have trouble getting to sleep. It is considered a far safer option than alcohol, which can put an individual to sleep, but which does not provide a deep, healthy sleep.

One major concern in using cannabis to improve sleep is that if and when you stop using cannabis, you may experience major withdrawals. As a result, ensure that you speak to your doctor about how much or how little cannabis you should use to avoid such issues.

Another major advantage of using CBD oil to help with sleep, is that lighter doses of CBD can keep the mind awake and the body active. As a result, you will not experience exhaustion or fatigue during the day and not feel the need to sleep during the day. This promotes good sleeping patterns and will encourage a deep sleep during the night.

One issue that comes with sleep is sleep apnea. Sleep apnea is a sleeping disorder that affects many Americans and that, if not treated, can lead to fatality. This disorder causes irregular breathing during sleep. This irregular breathing is caused by the airway narrowing and can cause immense distress. Having high blood pressure, being overweight, and having a larger neck are all ways for a person to develop sleep apnea.

Research has been conducted to determine if CBD can be effective in treating sleep apnea. As CBD can encourage deep sleep and reduce stress, it can significantly decrease the risks of and the symptoms associated with sleep apnea. Studies continue to be conducted on the effectiveness of CBD -- ensure you keep your eye out for new developments and consult your medical professional on their opinion about using CBD to treat sleep apnea.

Ease The Pain

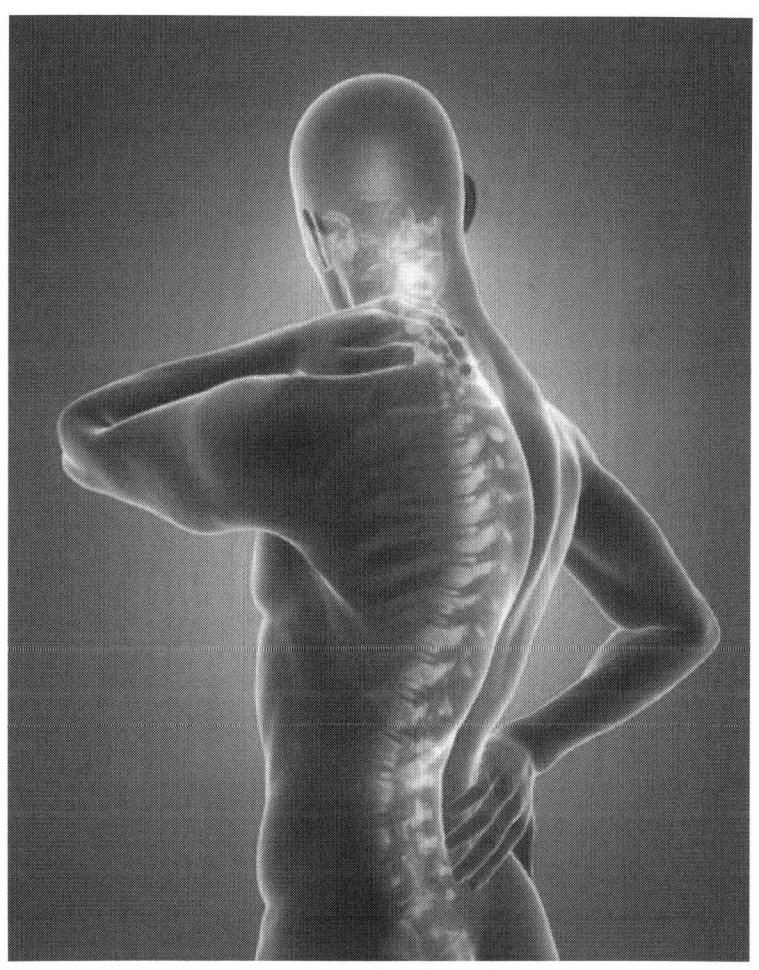

CBD oil has been used to treat a variety of body pains.

Image Credit: Shutterstock.com

I have discussed how CBD oil can be used to treat pain associated with rheumatoid arthritis. However, there are many other types of physical pain that can cause mild to severe discomfort and inconvenience. One of the most common forms of pain is back pain. As long as we continue to slouch over our desks and bury our noses in our smartphones, back pain will continue to be an issue. So, can you use CBD to treat back pain?

Studies have shown that low dosages have little effect on chronic back pain, but high doses were shown to ease the pain. To understand how CBD works against back pain, you need to understand how CBD affects the body in the first place. The human body and the brain contain serotonin, which is a neurotransmitter; vanilloid, which helps with stimuli such as feeling and touch; and adenosine, which focuses on physiological activity. As CBD is able to reduce inflammation, numb pain in the peripheral nervous system, and reduce stress, it is a great option for pain management.

Diabetes

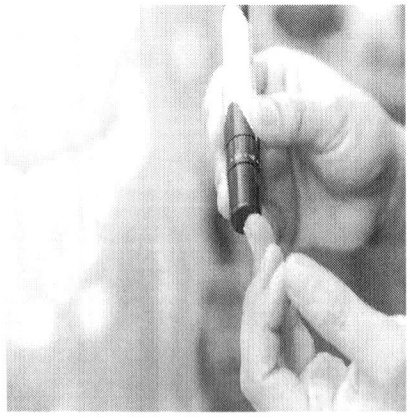

Diabetes is a common disease and affects individuals of all ages.

Image Credit: Shutterstock.com

There are two forms of diabetes: type 1 and type 2 diabetes. Type 1 diabetes arises when the beta cells, found in the pancreas, are destroyed. Beta cells are used to store insulin, which helps with building energy for the body. Type 2 diabetes includes a decrease in insulin, as well as high blood sugar levels. Regardless of type, diabetes is a difficult disease to deal with and there are many treatments available to combat the various symptoms. Research has been conducted to determine if cannabis can be used to treat diabetes.

This research has made the following observations in regard to CBD and diabetes:

1. CBD can control the high blood sugar levels associated with type 2 diabetes. One of the methods to *prevent* diabetes is to avoid high sugar foods or beverages. If you have high levels of sugar in your body, CBD can control these high levels.

2. CBD has an anti-inflammatory effect. Diabetes results in inflammation of the arteries and physicians often recommend an anti-inflammatory diet.. As CBD has anti-inflammatory properties, it can also be considered in the prevention and treatment of diabetes.

3. Particularly in type 2 diabetes, numbness or even pain can occur. As you have learned, CBD can be used for pain management and a person suffering from diabetes may use CBD to alleviate their pain in the same manner that someone with chronic back pain might.

4. Another symptom of diabetes is poor sleep. Furthermore, diabetes patients may feel excessively

fatigued. As previously discussed, CBD can awaken the body and the mind during the day and make sleep during the night more fulfilling and restful.

5. High blood pressure is a risk factor for many diseases, including diabetes. Increased and/or excessive activity of the nervous system can lead to high blood pressure; CBD can help the nervous system rest and relax.

Crohn's Disease

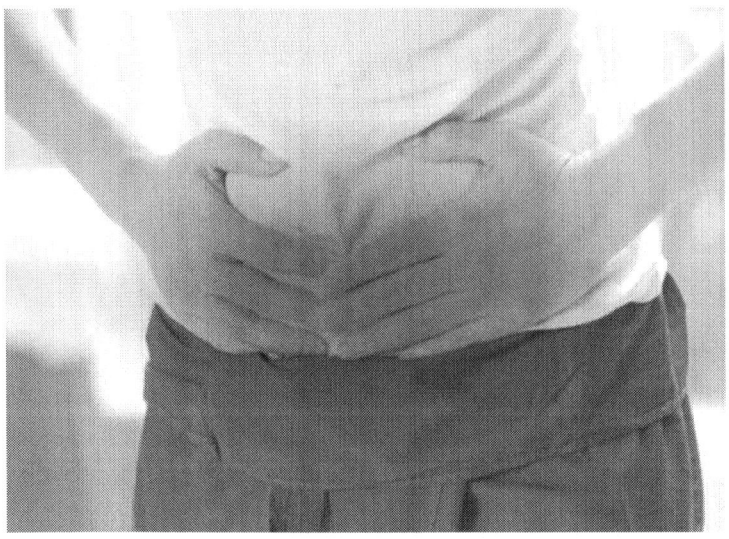

Crohn's disease is a bowel disease which can lead to abdominal pain, diarrhea, and weight loss.

Image Credit: Shutterstock.com

Crohn's disease is caused by inflammation of the bowels and can cause abdominal pain. Further symptoms include diarrhea and weight loss. It can even lead to inflammation of the eyes, fever, skin rashes, and exhaustion. As of this writing, the cause of Crohn's disease remains unknown; however, it is believed to be caused by exposure to an unhealthy environment, bacteria, and having a poor immune system. As of this writing, there is no cure for Crohn's disease, but there are many treatments to put the disease in remission and alleviate the suffering that comes with the symptoms.

Clinical trials on how CBD can treat inflammatory bowel diseases show good signs. As you have read, CBD provides anti-inflammatory effects. The endocannabinoid system is even found inside the gastrointestinal tract. These facts suggest that CBD is can help treat Crohn's disease. While studies on this subject are recent, there are already people who use CBD oil to treat their Crohn's disease. You should consult a medical professional before attempting this route to ensure that it is the best one for you.

Chapter Summary

- CBD oil has an incredible number of benefits for both physical and psychological disorders.

- This chapter is by no means a comprehensive list; more studies are being conducted on how CBD oil can treat other illnesses.

- CBD directly influences the endocannabinoid system.

In the next chapter, you will learn about what others say about the benefits of CBD oil.

Chapter Two: What Others Say

You have learned how CBD oil can help with various ailments in general terms, but the best way to learn about CBD oil and its benefits is to hear testimonials from those who have used it.

Doctors

Let us start with medical professionals. As of this writing, over 30 states, as well as the District of Columbia, have legalized the use of cannabis in some form -- mostly for medicinal purposes, with a few also allowing recreational use. Due to a court decision made in 2004, doctors may recommend the use of cannabis and its products, such as CBD oil, to their patients if they feel it can help with a patients' ailment.

Dr. Sanjay Gupta, once skeptical about cannabis, later changed his mind about the medicinal benefits of the plant. Cannabis has long been classified as a Schedule 1 drug by the Drug Enforcement Agency (DEA) in the United States. Dr. Gupta had been dismissive of many publications regarding the benefits of cannabis and took the side of the DEA. He eventually recanted this viewpoint and mentioned studies which shaped his new perspective.

In an article for CNN, Dr. Gupta writes about Charlotte Figi, who as a young child suffered from multiple seizures. Dr. Gupta describes how medicinal cannabis relaxed Charlotte's brain and lessened the number of seizures she would endure. He further writes on how a significant number of surveyed physicians would recommend medicinal cannabis to ease the pain of breast cancer.

Many other doctors have followed suit and advocated for medicinal cannabis. Dr. Joycelyn Elders, former Surgeon General for the United States, has been outspoken in her support for medicinal cannabis. She has long been an advocate for the legalization of marijuana and has spoken about how it has been used for thousands of years and should be used for medicinal purposes rather than suppressed.

Celebrities And Athletes

There have also been a number of celebrities who have endorsed the use of medicinal cannabis based on their personal experiences in using medicines such as CBD oil. Actress Whoopi Goldberg is one such person. She benefited from medicinal marijuana and decided to open her own dispensary along with business partner Maya Elisabeth. The focus of Whoopi & Maya is to produce cannabis products such as CBD oils to help with pain management and relief.

Former NFL quarterback Jake Plummer has joined with other football players to request the NFL open their policy on cannabis and consider hearing new research on the plant. Plummer has raised funds for research on how CBD can be used to treat grave diseases such as chronic traumatic encephalopathy (CTE), which is caused by repeated head injuries and is becoming commonplace in the NFL. Plummer himself has benefited from cannabis in several ways: he used it to alleviate the stress he felt from the game, and as the years progressed, he used it for pain relief. As he began to discover the benefits of cannabis use, he became active in increasing awareness of its' benefits and urging further research be conducted.

Plummer is not the only football player to advocate for cannabis use. Former NFL running back Ricky Williams was suspended in 2006 for using cannabis. In spite of the backlash he received, he has gone on record to state that he does not regret his cannabis use. He has been vocal about how the plant has helped him improve his overall wellness.

Everyday People

Although it is comforting to hear that medical professionals recognize the benefits of cannabis and CBD oil and that well-known celebrities and athletes advocate for its use, perhaps the best way to convince you to move past your skepticism is to share testimonials from people just like you.

Noah Novello suffered from herniated discs after being injured at work. He was prescribed a multitude of pills which not only did not ease the pain, but left him with several undesirable side effects. However, with the first application of CBD oil, Noah immediately felt the pain significantly decrease.

Another incredible success story is from Kendra Cochran, who had her hand cut open by a glass bottle. The pain was intense and the prescription painkillers did nothing to alleviate the pain. To make matters worse, they increased her discomfort and made her nauseous. CBD oil was the thing that helped Kendra cope with her pain.

In the previous chapter, you learned how CBD oil can be used to treat acne. However, acne is not the only skin disease which can be treated with CBD oil. Steven Daniels suffers from a rare skin disease called Hailey-Hailey. This disease causes blisters to develop all over the skin and can be extremely painful. With Hailey-Hailey, patients are normally prescribed steroids which do even greater harm by weakening the skin. Steven used a CBD ointment to fight bacteria and keep his condition under control.

Jason Burruss had difficulty experiencing deep sleep. He would sleep at late hours and wake up frequently during the night. CBD has helped him experience deep sleep and wake up feeling energized.

Shannon Donnelly has an extreme form of anxiety and, in the past, often suffered from panic attacks. To make matters worse, she would feel depressed and have suicidal thoughts. CBD helped Shannon feel more confident and comfortable in various situations.

The above stories were taken from <u>CBD Success Stories: How Cannabidiol Improves Lives</u> *from Westword.com*

The serious study of CBD and hemp oils for medicinal use began once these and other success stories began to garner mass attention. I would highly recommend that you familiarize yourself with as many success stories as you can to improve your understanding of the benefits of medicinal cannabis and for CBD and hemp products. Many of these stories can be found on the Internet, in magazines and journals, and even in books. Although we do not have time to cover them all here, these relevant examples should give you a taste of what is out there.

Here's one last story that prompted much attention from the scientific community. Although there was no use of cannabis or CBD oil and this is not a success story per se, this incident did spark a flurry of cannabis research.

In late 2017, a man woke up from a coma which he had been in for fifteen years! This, of course, was a joyous occasion, but it also resulted in many questions from doctors and researchers. Those who studied the man concluded that the vagus nerve, considered one of the most important nerves in the body, can help restore brain function and probably helped the coma patient regain consciousness.

But wait. What about this situation could possibly have prompted researchers to study cannabis? Hold on and you'll see. One of the stereotypes we have regarding cannabis is that its users often get the "munchies" and eat whatever food they can find. This is because cannabis reacts with the digestive tract. And what, you might ask, does that have to do with our coma patient? The vagus nerve, cited as a factor in his recovery, is connected to the digestive tract. In fact, an article in *Cannabis and Cannabinoid Research* confirms that cannabis stimulates the vagus nerve.

Although cannabis did not play a role in this particular coma patient's recovery, scientists quickly made the link between the role played by the vagus nerve in his recovery and cannabis's effect on the vagus nerve. This led to an increase in research on the benefits of cannabis and its products, like CBD oil

.As you can see, the openness toward using CBD has increased tremendously, because of both scientific research and real-life testimonials. As more success stories emerge, more and more people support the use (at least medicinally) of cannabis and CBD oil. How could they not, when it has brought such great relief to so many? Who knows? If you implement a CBD oil regimen in your life, and you could become the next success story!

Chapter Summary

- As researchers have discovered new information about the benefits and uses of cannabis, more physicians have opened their minds to CBD use.

- CBD is supported by celebrities and everyday people who have used it and found that it relieved their ailments, ranging from skin diseases to seizures.

- With more success stories comes more support for research.

In the next chapter, you will learn about hemp oil and its benefits.

Chapter Three: Hemp Oil

I have discussed in great length the benefits of CBD oil. In this chapter, I want to briefly introduce you to a topic which will complement your knowledge of CBD oil: hemp oil. While CBD oil is extracted from the cannabis plant, hemp oil is developed by pressing hemp seeds. Hemp oils range from a light to a dark color, with the latter having a more grass-type flavor and the former having a nut-type flavor. Hemp oil can also be refined, although with this procedure it loses all of its nutritional value. This type of hemp oil is used for many everyday products but does not carry medicinal value.

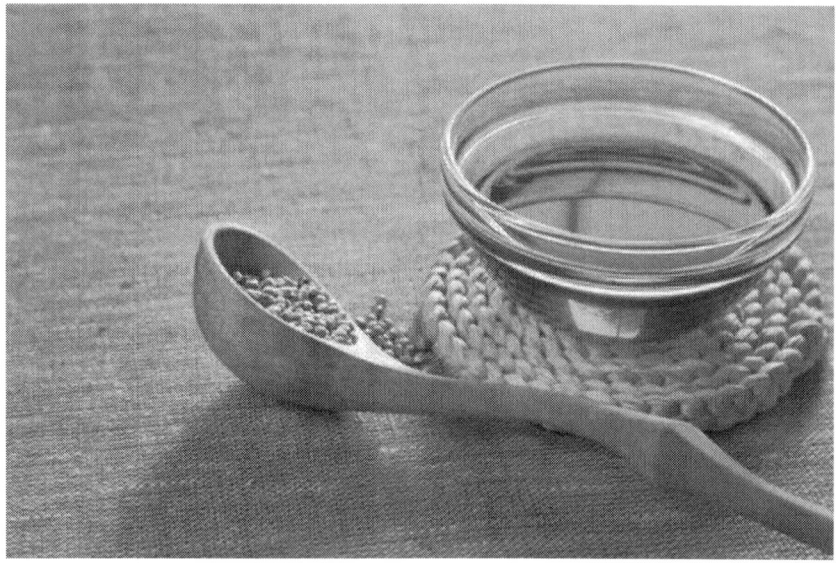

Hemp seeds and hemp oil have practical, nutritional, and medicinal value.

Image Credit: Shutterstock.com

Hemp oil is often used for cooking and as a supplement to one's diet because of its nutritional and medicinal value. There are three key components that give hemp seeds their value:

1. They contain *essential fatty acids*. Essential fatty acids are needed to fuel and energize the body. Physicians recommend a diet that is rich in essential fatty acids, but it is often difficult to consume the recommended amount. Think about how much protein is recommended from your diet and how much easier it is to consume this protein if at least a portion of it is consumed through a protein shake. Hemp oil contains omega-3 and omega-6 fatty acids, which have a breadth of benefits.

    a. Omega-3 fatty acids can lower the concentration of triglycerides (fat) in the blood, which is essential for preventing and lowering the risk of heart disease.

    b. Omega-3 fatty acids also play a role in anti-inflammation which you know by now is essential for overall wellness and can help with alleviating pain.

    c. Omega-3 fatty acids have also been found to fight depression.

    d. Omega-6 fatty acids help with cell growth. This is crucial for developing both the brain and the muscles. It is no surprise that omega-6 is often found in foods with a high protein content.

2. Hemp oil is rich in *linoleic acids.*

    a. Linoleic acids are full of antioxidants, which can expunge free radicals. Free radicals, while having benefits to the human body, can also be a danger and have been linked to Parkinson's disease, schizophrenia, and even Alzheimer's disease.

    b. Linoleic acids are the main factor in fighting heart disease.

3. Hemp oil is also high in *vitamin E*.

    a. Vitamin E is plentiful in many North American diets and is found in a range of foods, from corn oil to margarine.

    b. Like linoleic acids, vitamin E is a great antioxidant.

    c. On average, each 100 grams of hemp seeds can have between 6 (whole seeds) and 8 (hulled Seeds or nuts) milligrams of vitamin E. The daily recommendation in the United States is 15 milligrams.

    d. Finally, vitamin E is lauded as an anti-aging supplement. Wrinkles, stretch marks, and other blemishes are to be expected as one gets older. However, a healthy dose of vitamin E can conceal these age-showing blemishes.

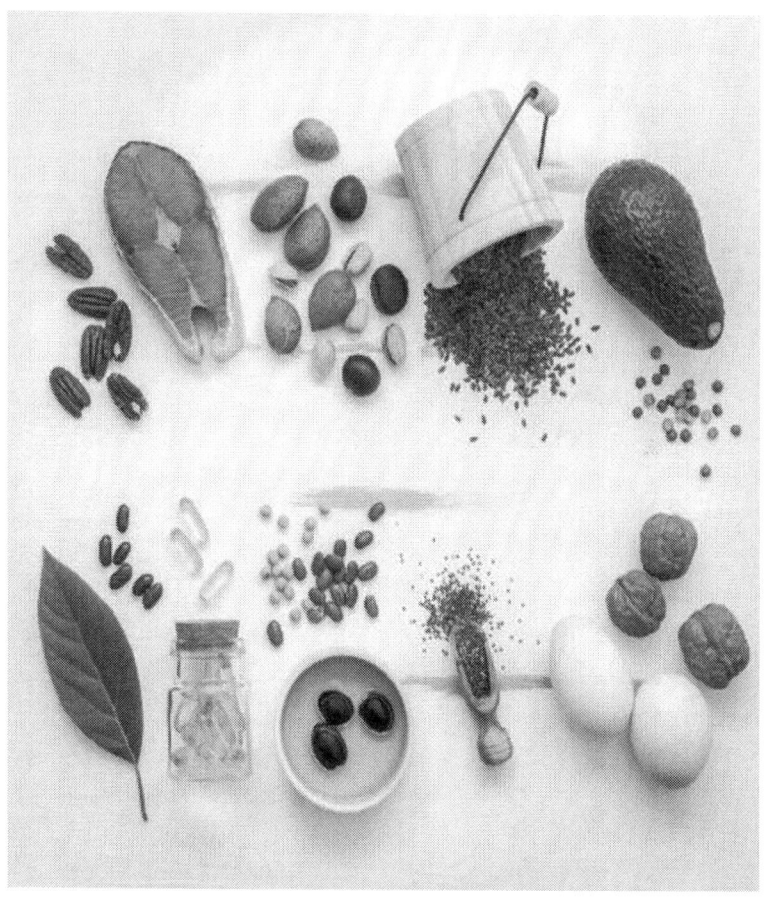

Eggs, avocados, and nuts contain the same nutrients found in hemp seeds and hemp oil.

Image Credit: Shutterstock.com

Like CBD oil, hemp oil can come in a variety of forms.

For example, hemp oil can be used as a lotion. It contains components which are beneficial to one's skin -- in particular, vitamin E. As a lotion, hemp can improve skin-tissue growth and encourage skin elasticity. It can also decrease skin flaking and even help with the treatment of acne, just as CBD oil can.

One of the most popular uses of hemp oil is in the kitchen. You can use hemp oil as an alternative to the usual vegetable or olive oil used in cooking. As hemp seeds produce a nutty taste, using hemp oil to cook can add this flavor to your food. You can even use it as a salad dressing or for dipping bread. Some culinary enthusiasts even recommend incorporating it into a sauce such as hummus or mayonnaise. As hemp oil is rich in essential fatty acids, linoleic acids, and vitamin E, there is every reason to use it in your cooking.

So, now we know that hemp oil is rich in nutrients and can be extremely beneficial to your overall wellness. But the big question is: has hemp oil met with the same success as CBD oil?

Of particular note is one story about how hemp oil turned things around for a two-year-old child named Silas Algire. Silas suffered from epilepsy. Epilepsy is a disorder which leads to seizures. Seizures are characterized by the body convulsing intensely, and may even lead to the individual losing consciousness. This is a frightening prospect for anyone, but it is particularly frightening for a child as young as two years of age.

Even after using the often prescribed Trileptal, Silas's seizures did not cease and he was frequently fussy, according to his mother Kiana. After being introduced to CBD oil and hemp oil, Silas's seizures began to lessen and have now ceased. Originally, Kiana did not understand why so many patients refused to take medicines recommended by physicians. However, she now realizes that these medications may be ineffective and can even cause damage to the body. Hemp oil does not present side effects in most patients, and in the case of Silas, it was the best medicine for his recovery.

Hemp oil may be a great option for treating an illness or for use as a supplement to improve your general wellness. Ask your physician if they recommend hemp oil and consider using it if you are given the go ahead!

As a final note, you may be wondering how hemp oil compares to CBD oil and which one is "better." Neither is necessarily better, though one may be more beneficial to you depending on your needs and how you would like to use your oil. Here are the essential differences between the two:

1. Hemp oil is derived from hemp seeds; CBD oil is derived directly from the stalk of the cannabis plant.

2. Hemp oil contains essential fatty acids and related nutrients; CBD oil contains cannabinoids, terpenoids, and flavonoids.

3. CBD oil can directly affect the endocannabinoid system. One benefit is that it can numb aches and pains. Hemp oil is more adept at providing your body with essential nutrients for health and wellness.

Chapter Summary

- Hemp oil contains essential fatty acids, linoleic acids, and vitamin E, which can all be found in food, but which can be difficult to get enough of.

- Hemp oil can be used in your food and can be used to cook with.

In the next chapter, you will learn how to determine which product is right for you.

Chapter Four: Which Is For Me?

So, now that you know all about CBD and hemp oils, including their benefits and how they are different, you have decided to try one (or both) of them and incorporate it into your life. This brings up a new question: *Which is the right product for me?*

Your medical professional will know best what is best-suited for your current health condition as well as your goals. However, knowing the similarities and differences between the two is important so that your consultation is a conversation in which you can provide educated reasoning and questions.

The unique aspect of CBD oil is that it contains CBD (obviously!). As you have learned, CBD has many benefits and can serve as a treatment to many illnesses. These benefits include anti-inflammation, relaxing the mind, and strengthening the joints. The components of hemp oil are essential fatty acids, linoleic acid, and vitamin E -- which can all be found elsewhere. This may make you feel that CBD oil is the way to go and that hemp oil is unnecessary. However, it may be easier for you to get them from using hemp oil in your cooking or taking is as a supplement than absorbing them from whole food sources.

CBD also directly affects the body's endocannabinoid system, which is especially helpful if you wish to tackle psychological disorders such as anxiety and depression. Hemp oil does not affect the endocannabinoid system and is more suited for tackling physical health issues. In short, both oils can be used for overall wellness, but CBD oil has the additional advantage of treating psychological disorders and more severe illnesses.

In the United States, CBD oil is legal in all states only on the condition that it is industrialized. This means that the end product is the result of industrial production. There are several methods of this:

CO_2

The CBD oil is extracted from the cannabis plant by adding pressurized carbon dioxide to act as a solvent and produce the desired result. This is the most expensive method, but it is the method that ensures the best quality of CBD oil product. Because of this, I would recommend that you only purchase CBD oil that is produced through this method.

Carrier Oil

This is also known as the "olive oil method." The cannabis plant is heated and then mixed with the carrier oil. This mixture is heated to a very high temperature (248 degrees Fahrenheit) so the cannabinoids can be extracted from the plant. The final product is a mixture which contains the carrier oil. This method is especially helpful if using CBD on your skin as opposed to ingesting it.

Solvents

This method requires the plant to be mixed with ethanol, butane, or a low-grade alcohol. The mixed solvent will extract the cannabinoids and once the liquid is heated, the solvent will evaporate and leave behind the final CBD oil product. This is ideal if your preferred method for consuming CBD is vaping.

So, what about hemp oil? As you have read, there are two types of hemp oil -- one that is light in color and one that is dark in color. For topical purposes (applying oil to the skin) you may want to opt for a hemp oil that is light in color. This type of hemp oil has been refined and is used in many beauty products. Otherwise, hemp oil is normally cold-pressed and appears dark in color. This is the type of hemp oil that has the nutty or earthy flavor and retains its nutritional value.

You now know the differences between the two types of oil and how they are developed. Here is a quick exercise I recommend. On a piece of paper, answer the following questions. Once you have an idea of what you really want from CBD and/or hemp oil, you will be able to communicate your goals to your medical professional, who can advise you.

1. What are the illnesses or disorders you have which you wish to treat? What are the illnesses or disorders which you wish to prevent?

2. What changes to your diet (if any) would you like to make? If you feel your diet is fine, what needs to be maintained to sustain your good health?

3. How often would you like to incorporate medicinal cannabis into your life? Would you want to use CBD or hemp oil on a daily basis? On a weekly basis? Or just once in a blue moon?

4. What is your preferred way of consuming the medicinal cannabis product? What would be the most convenient (and enjoyable) method for you to consume the product?

5. How mild or severe are your ailments or how bad is your overall health that you feel you need to use

medicinal cannabis? Be honest, as this will help determine the appropriate dosage and the best method for consuming the product, as well as whether you should use a CBD product, a hemp product, or both!

Chapter Summary

- Hemp oil works best as a supplement to your diet. CBD oil is a standalone treatment.

- CBD oil effects your endocannabinoid system, while hemp oil does not. If your issue is psychological, CBD oil is a better choice.

- Determine your needs to decide which product is better for you.

In the next chapter, you will learn about how to purchase and consume CBD oil and hemp oil.

Chapter Five: How To Get It

The question you most likely have now is two-fold: *Where do I purchase CBD oil? And how exactly should I consume it?*

In this case, it is best to answer the second question first. There are a number of ways to consume CBD oil:

1. The simplest and most-preferred method is straight CBD oil. Probably the greatest benefit of CBD oil is that it can be used as an ingredient alongside almost any edible. You can add it to your morning smoothie, incorporate it into brownies or cookies, or even take it plain as you would any liquid medicine.

2. Another popular option is a CBD tincture. A tincture is an extract of CBD and comes in a small bottle with a dropper to absorb and release the liquid. Like a CBD oil, a CBD tincture can be consumed as is or by mixing with an edible or other liquid. With the dropper, you can more precisely measure the amount of CBD to consume. If you (or your physician) feel that your dosage needs to be precise, this is the best option for you.

3. Applying cannabis directly to the human skin has been a practice for many years. CBD topicals come in many forms: ointments, lotions, creams, balms, and salves. If you are using CBD to ease pain in your muscles or joints or to treat any skin conditions, opting for a CBD topical may be your best bet.

4. Vaping is another popular option for consuming CBD oil. Vaping has become a popular alternative to

smoking tobacco and in the case of cannabis, the advantage of vaping is that it allows the individual to absorb the benefits of CBD without worrying about the side effects of throat or lung irritation. For vaping, the CBD oil is generally combined with another liquid to allow the CBD to be absorbed easily. Often vaporizers will come in a variety of flavors to enhance the experience of consumption.

5. Like CBD tinctures, CBD sublingual sprays can be used for precise measurement of doses. These sprays are intended to be sprayed under your tongue. If you need a precise amount of CBD and want to absorb it as quickly as possible without having to go through the fuss of mixing it with edibles or liquids, then sublingual sprays are the best route to take!

You may be unsure of what method to use. Do you opt in for an oil or an ointment? CBD or hemp? Both? As always, your medical professional will be able to provide you with the best advice. Do what is most comfortable to you and discuss the various options available with your doctor. Ask them about the advantages and disadvantages of choosing one type of product over another.

How To Shop

When it comes to purchasing CBD or hemp oil at a store or online, there is good and bad news. The good news is that there are many retailers and brands which sell these oils in abundance. The bad news is that there many retailers and brands which sell these oils in abundance! Before purchasing CBD or hemp products, it is essential that you conduct your research and develop a sense of discernment to figure out what are the best options for you and what products to avoid altogether.

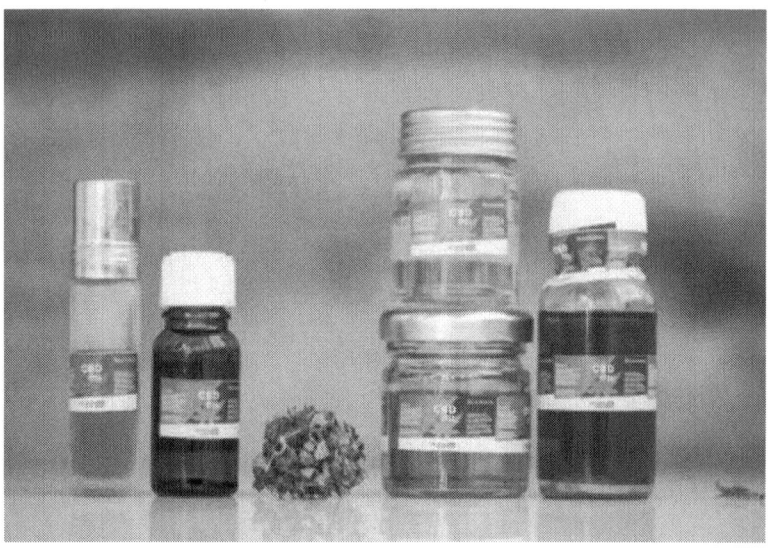

When purchasing CBD products, inspect the labels to ensure they are self-regulated and meet accepted guidelines. Ask your medical professional for the brands they suggest.

Image Credit: Shutterstock.com

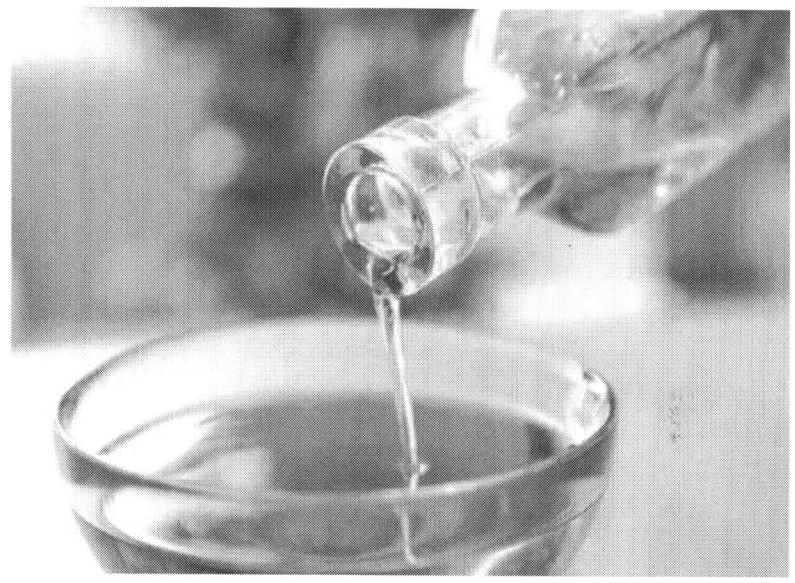

Wait! Before you add hemp oil to your cooking, ensure that it also meets the accepted guidelines and standards. Ask your medical professional what brand of hemp oil they suggest.

Image Credit: Shutterstock.com

The DEA has kept its eye on the market to ensure that no illegal or harmful CBD or hemp products are distributed. You will have to know what products are not only legal but also safe and effective to use. For purchasing CBD products, ensure that they meet ALL three of the following criteria:

> 1. Lab results from an impartial source. Ensure that studies regarding the product are published and easily accessible. They must be from a credible source that does not have an agenda. Simply seeing several positive reviews from consumers is insufficient -- you want to buy products that have been endorsed by top researchers, scientists, and medical professionals.

2. Ensure that the product is made using the CO2 extraction process. You want to ensure that when CBD or hemp is extracted, it is done without any interference or mixing of another chemical which may be left behind in the final product and could cause you harm.

3. As you have learned, the key difference between marijuana and cannabidiol is the level of THC. Remember that THC is what causes the psychoactive effects associated with smoking marijuana. You want to make sure that the CBD and hemp products you consume have a concentration of THC *less* than 0.3%.

As of this writing, one of the top selling brands in the United States is Medix CBD. You should consider this a good brand to start with, but, as always, please conduct extensive research when choosing a brand and consult a medical professional to decide which brand or brands to settle on before you make a purchase.

It is understandable that you may be on a tight budget, but it is imperative not to opt for the cheapest option. Ensure that the manufacturers of the products regulate their own products and provide detailed verification that their products meet the guidelines listed previously.

As of this writing, the legal cannabis industry within the United States is unregulated. This poses many problems -- the consumer will not know what the best and safest products to purchase are. This book is here to ensure that you are a smart and informed consumer and I encourage you to pass this information to others so that we can create a culture of informed CBD and hemp consumers.

Chapter Summary

- At present, the legal cannabis industry is unregulated. This necessitates that you do your research and be smart about the products you choose to use.

- Follow the guidelines set forth by the DEA so that you purchase the best quality and safest products.

- Always consult a medical professional before making a purchase.

In the next chapter, you will learn more details about the legality of CBD and hemp oils and of cannabis in general.

Chapter Six: Legal Information

By now, you are probably eager to try out CBD and/or hemp products to improve your health conditions and your overall wellness. But there is still one more major hurdle to cross: *Is this even legal?*

This is a fair question and the answer is quite complex. You must ensure that the product you choose falls within the realm of *legal cannabis use*. As of this writing, medicinal cannabis is legal in all 50 states in the United States. However, as previously mentioned, the market is currently NOT under regulation by the Food and Drug Administration (FDA).

Here are some general guidelines to follow to ensure the legality of a CBD or hemp product:

1. Ensure that there is verifiable information printed on the package that meets the guidelines discussed in the previous chapter.

2. Ensure that the material is pure and not mixed with any extraneous materials which could cause harm. There should be no added chemicals. Consult your medical professional on what materials/ingredients could fall under this purview.

3. Ensure that the products are rich in cannabinoids. The products must be low in THC (remember 0.3%) to differentiate it from recreational marijuana, which remains *illegal* in many states.

At this point, it would be prudent to learn some legal background and discuss how far cannabis has come from in terms of legality.

The 1936 film *Reefer Madness* was made to warn parents about the dangers of their children smoking cannabis. Today, it is lampooned and viewed as a comedic film as opposed to a serious tale of moral degradation as was the film's intention. That is because the knowledge regarding the effects of cannabis are considerably more sophisticated today than they were in 1936.

Ensure that you check your state (in some cases, even your city or town) laws on the legality of purchasing a CBD and/or hemp oil. In many states, CBD that comes directly from the cannabis plant is NOT legal, since there may be a higher percentage of THC than is permitted. If this is the case in your area, you would have to purchase CBD that is produced synthetically. If the CBD is derived from industrial hemp, it will have the permitted percentage of THC.

In Chapter Two, you learned briefly about Charlotte Figi and how her case has been instrumental in increasing awareness of the medicinal value of cannabis. Another story which was even more instrumental in pushing for legalization is the story of Cash Hyde. Like Charlotte, Cash suffered from a grave illness at a young age. Cash had a tumor, and radiation and traditional treatments were not improving his condition. Although it was in violation of the laws of Montana, Cash's father, Mike, gave his toddler cannabis oil to treat the tumor. The cannabis oil seemed to work, as Cash remained alive for slightly over two years afterward. He sadly passed away when access to cannabis oil became even more restricted by the laws of Montana. However, many medical professionals praised Mike Hyde for providing his son with the cannabis oil and discussions regarding the benefits and the proposed legalization of medicinal cannabis were underway.

While no consensus exists and many medical professionals "recommend" as opposed to "prescribe" any form of medicinal cannabis, there are constantly new developments. By the time you read this, there may be states where prescribed cannabis has become commonplace. Whether or not that is the case, one good thing is that research regarding the medicinal value of cannabis is now taken seriously and many people have accepted the benefits of it as fact. The fact that you can easily access the information found in this book means that we are much closer to widespread acceptance than even just a few years ago.

Of course, the history of cannabis is a long one. In ancient China and India, the cannabis plant was used for both medicinal and recreational purposes. Slowly, the plant found its way to North Africa and, after many years, eventually made it to the Americas and what is now the United States. Prior to cotton, hemp was a popular crop that was harvested in the Southern United States. In the 1920s, it became even more popular as it was smoked as marijuana. Surprisingly, it was not taboo at the time, and though it was used for recreational purposes, it was also used for medicinal purposes. In the early 1940s, it was used as a treatment for different types of pains. While it had its critics who classified it as a "gateway drug" to more dangerous drugs, it continued to flourish well into the 1950s and 1960s when it became the drug of choice for the hippie generation. However, in the 1970s, marijuana was classified as a Schedule I drug -- meaning that it was considered one of the most dangerous drugs (along with heroin and cocaine) and had *no medicinal value*!

That attitude and stigma toward cannabis -- based in untruth -- is what is being fought against, and success stories within the last decade and serious research on the medical benefits of CBD and hemp are slowly but surely washing away this stigma. The DEA remains stringent on their perspective that cannabis is a dangerous drug. There have been movements to request (or demand!) the DEA "de-schedule" cannabis, and while this has been to no avail, there is support from some members of the U.S. government for the medicinal and, in some cases, recreational use of cannabis.

As the laws continue to change, ensure that you are up-to-date with the laws in your area. The good news is that as of this writing, you can purchase CBD and hemp oils regardless of what area of the United States you live in as long as they contain little to no THC. As always, ensure you follow the current guidelines, keep up with developments, and seek the advice of a medical professional before taking any new CBD or hemp product.

Chapter Summary

- Attitudes toward cannabis have changed over time.

- Check your state's laws regarding the finer points of the legality of cannabis.

- With continued research, the stigma is slowly fading away.

In the next chapter, you will learn how to continue your wellness journey using CBD and/or hemp Oil.

Wellness

One must remember that wellness is a continuous journey. Even if you feel that you are in good health and do not suffer from any ailments, your body and mind must ALWAYS be maintained. The medicinal components of CBD and hemp can help you in your quest to maintain your overall health. One of the ways to continue on this path is to ensure you are always knowledgeable about CBD and hemp and any new developments. Refer to this last chapter every now and then as a way to develop discipline in looking after your health.

Let *us take a moment to recap the lessons you have learned:

1. The Cannabis plant has been used for centuries and across civilizations for recreational purposes -- but more importantly, for medicinal purposes.

2. The medicinal purposes range from treating bodily pains to treating psychological disorders to helping with the most serious of illnesses such as cancer or CTE.

3. CBD is extracted from the stalk of the cannabis plant and can be consumed in a variety of forms: as an oil, capsule, tincture, suppository, chewing gum, ointment, sublingual spray, etc.

4. Hemp oil is derived from the hemp seeds themselves. The oil has a nutty flavor and can be light green to dark green in color.

5. CBD affects the cannabinoid receptors of the endocannabinoid system and, as a result, can have effects ranging from easing physical pain to relaxing the mind.

6. As we see more and more success stories, medicinal cannabis is being taken more seriously. Research into the benefits of CBD and hemp products continues to flourish.

7. In the United States, the market is currently unregulated. As a result, you may come across some subpar products. As always, conduct your research before purchasing a product and always speak to a medical professional so they can determine what is best for you.

Now, ask yourself these questions and provide the answers. Try not to cheat by looking back in the book! Answer to the best of your abilities and then look back to see what you got correct and understood and what still needs grasping. Do not worry about scoring. Your wellness is a continued journey and there is always more to learn.

1. CBD oil and hemp oil produce the same psychoactive effects as smoking marijuana. True or False?

2. CBD oil and hemp oil are essentially the same. They both treat the same ailments in the same manner and, therefore, it does not matter which one you purchase, right? WRONG, OF COURSE! Write down your best explanation of the differences between the two and how they can benefit your wellness in different ways.

3. What are the different methods of taking CBD and why would you choose one over the other?

4. Brainstorm how you would incorporate hemp oil into your diet.

5. Hemp oil contains essential fatty acids, linoleic acid, and vitamin E. What benefits do each of these components have?

6. How can CBD oil treat: acne, diabetes, back pain, Crohn's disease, depression, and anxiety? Apart from what you have read in this book, have you read any studies on CBD oil treating a different ailment?

7. Apart from what you have read in this book, are there any success stories you know of or have studied relating to CBD and/or hemp? Document and record these continuously.

Make sure you look back at these questions and revise your answers to the last two questions every now and then. You have read this book because you were curious about how CBD and Hemp Oil could benefit your health. However, I want you to think of this book not only as a source of information, but also as a guide which you will follow to maintain a healthy lifestyle using CBD and/or hemp products.

Conclusion

By now, I can confidently say that you are more knowledgeable about medicinal cannabis than before. You should be less skeptical about the medicinal value of this plant and more open to implementing CBD and hemp products in your life to treat any ailments and promote your overall wellness . Thank you for reading this book! I wish you luck on your journey to health and happiness!

If you found this book helpful please leave a positive review on Amazon as it is greatly appreciated and keeps me being able to deliver high quality books.

Made in the USA
Lexington, KY
03 November 2018